YOUR PATH TO A HEALTHIER YOU

LOSE WEIGHT, BEAT OBESITY

ANNE C. CHESHIRE

TABLE OF CONTENTS

INTRODUCTION

Matilda had battled obesity ever since she was a young adult. Since she was young, she had struggled with being overweight and several health issues, such as type 2 diabetes, high blood pressure, and high cholesterol. She tried her hardest to adjust her lifestyle, but she couldn't keep the weight off.

When Matilda finally lost it, she made the decision to act. She started looking into weight-loss methods and came across a diet and exercise regimen that was successful for her. She also used the assistance of nutritionists, counselors, and medical professionals to help her stay on track.

It was not an easy road for Matilda to lose weight. Yet she was finally able to fulfill her goal of decreasing weight and leading a healthier life with devotion, perseverance, and hard work.

The tactics Matilda employed to overcome her difficulties with obesity are detailed in this book. She will talk about her physical, mental, and emotional struggles as well as how she overcame them. Also, Matilda will share advice on how to maintain an active lifestyle, eat well, and create a positive body image.

The story of Matilda's journey is one of optimism and tenacity. Her experience might encourage people who are having difficulty losing weight and serve as a motivating example for those who doubt their own abilities

This book is a motivational and educational resource for combating obesity. Our objective is that it will empower people to take charge of their lives and improve their health and happiness.

CHAPTER 1

WHAT IS OBESITY?

Definition: Obesity, sometimes referred to as corpulence or fatness, is the excessive buildup of bodily fat, typically brought on by consuming more calories than the body can utilize. The extra calories are subsequently turned into fat, also known as adipose tissue. Particularly in people with large or muscular bones, moderate weight gain does not always equate to obesity.

The previous definition of obesity was a rise in body weight that was greater than 20% of a person's optimal body weight, which was the weight associated with the lowest risk of death based on characteristics like age, height, and gender. Hence, a 15–20% rise over optimal body weight might be used to diagnose overweight based on the aforementioned criteria. Yet, today's definitions of obesity and overweight are mostly based on weight and height measurements rather than morbidity.

A value known as the body mass index (BMI) is computed using these measurements. This figure, which is crucial for assessing whether a person is clinically characterized as obese, mirrors fatness but does not directly reflect body fat. Based on weight status classifications, such as underweight, healthy weight, overweight, and obese, which are adjusted for age and sex, BMI values are understood. BMI values are used to categorize weight status for all adults over the age of 20; for example, a BMI between 25.0 and 29.9 is considered to be overweight, and a BMI of 30.0 or more is considered to be obese. A BMI of 40.0 or more is deemed to be morbid obesity (sometimes referred to as extreme, severe, or other forms of obesity).

Obesity Factors

Activity and food:

Obesity is largely caused by food and activity. Weight gain can result from consuming an excessive amount of unhealthy foods, such as processed snacks, fast food, and junk food. These foods tend to be high in calories, fat, and sugar, which can cause weight gain. Nevertheless, obesity can also be a result of insufficient physical activity.

Because of a slowed metabolism brought on by inactivity, the body may begin to accumulate more calories and fat. A person may find it difficult to move and stay active if they don't exercise because of a loss in strength and muscular mass. A person's risk of being obese can be decreased by choosing healthier foods and engaging in more physical activity.

Environment:

Obesity, particularly in children, is now commonly acknowledged to have environmental causes. Unprecedented environmental changes, both natural and man-made, brought on by our contemporary lives are seriously affecting our health and wellbeing. Several environmental changes may affect the prevalence of obesity directly or indirectly.

Influences from the environment can boost calorie intake directly. This is brought on by the accessibility of calorie-dense foods that frequently have low nutritional value and the encouragement of sedentary lifestyles. Due to their increased likelihood of being exposed to unhealthy food and beverage promotions, children are especially at risk. The architectural layout of our cities, or the built environment, can also limit access to chances for physical activity and promote sedentary behavior.

Environmental elements, including air pollution, climate change, and socioeconomic inequality, can all indirectly cause obesity. The endocrine system can be upset by air pollution, which also causes an increase in fat storage. Extreme weather events brought on by climate change might impede the flow of food through supply networks, resulting in hunger and undernutrition. Socioeconomic gaps can also result in a lack of access to options for a healthy diet and physical activity.

It is obvious that the environment is a crucial consideration.

Genetics:

A number of variables, including genetic predisposition, contribute to the complicated medical disease known as obesity. Because specific genetic variants may affect hunger, metabolism, and fat storage, it is thought that genetics may play a part in obesity.

Given the high hereditary component of obesity, certain people may be predisposed to the disease due to specific genetic factors. Both parents may contribute to the inheritance of these genes, which may be passed down through the generations. Moreover, environmental elements, including diet, exercise habits, and lifestyle choices, might interact with these genes to raise a person's risk of obesity.

For instance, some people may have a gene that increases their propensity to accumulate fat in their abdomen region, raising their chance of becoming obese. Some people may have a genotype that makes them more inclined to react to hormones that stimulate appetite and cravings. Additionally, some people may have genes that increase their likelihood of being less active and burning fewer calories, which elevates their risk of obesity.

There is no single "obesity gene," and the relationship between genetics and environment can be complex.

Medical conditions and treatments: Obesity is a major medical disease that impacts millions of individuals globally. It is frequently related to living an unhealthy lifestyle, which includes eating poorly and doing little exercise. Obesity, however, can also be caused by a wide range of additional variables, such as medical disorders and drugs.

Some medical diseases, such as hypothyroidism, polycystic ovarian syndrome, and Cushing's disease, can cause weight gain. Certain ailments may trigger the body to create hormones that impact metabolism and result in weight gain.

Weight gain might also result from taking some drugs. Weight gain may be a side effect of several antipsychotics, birth control pills, and antidepressants. A few drugs used to treat diabetes, high blood pressure, and high cholesterol might also make you gain weight.

Finally, some lifestyle choices might also result in weight gain. For instance, the body's normal hormone balance can be disturbed by stress, lack of sleep, and some drugs, which can result in weight gain.

It's critical to realize that obesity is a complex disorder with a variety of causes. Healthy food and regular exercise are crucial for keeping a healthy weight, but it's also important to be aware of any diseases or drugs that could cause weight gain. See your doctor about your health and any drugs you are taking if you are worried about your weight.

Stress: Stress has been linked to the emergence of obesity more and more frequently. Overeating and insufficient exercise are two harmful behaviors that are frequently associated with stress. According to theory, comfort food cravings are triggered by stress chemicals like cortisol. Obesity and weight gain can result from overeating in response to stress.

Moreover, stress might cause the formation of bad behaviors that support obesity. For instance, stressed-out people could find themselves skipping meals or indulging in unhealthy snacks as a coping mechanism. In addition to causing changes in sleep habits, stress can also affect how much you weigh. Lack of sleep can cause weight gain and obesity by increasing appetite and decreasing physical activity.

Last but not least, stress can alter the gut microbiota, which can directly affect weight. The energy balance and metabolism, both of which can be impacted by stress, are believed to be influenced by the gut flora.

All things considered, stress may have a role in the onset of obesity. To keep a healthy weight, it's critical to understand how stress affects you and develop coping mechanisms.

Low sleep quality:

An important contributing factor to the rise in obesity is now more widely acknowledged to be poor sleep. Insufficient sleep can result in sedentary lifestyles and bad eating habits, both of which are primary causes of obesity.

Lack of sleep can make you feel fatigued and exhausted, which might make you unmotivated to work out and be physically active. As a result, the number of calories burned may drop, which could result in an increase in body fat storage.

In addition to disrupting the circadian cycle of the body, poor sleep can also affect the levels of the hunger hormones leptin and ghrelin. Leptin and ghrelin are two hormones that affect satiety, while ghrelin is a hormone that increases hunger. These hormones can become out of balance, which can increase appetite and cravings for unhealthy foods, which can lead to overeating and an increase in body fat reserves.

Cortisol and other stress hormones can rise as a result of inadequate sleep. Increased fat storage and cravings for fatty and sugary foods are two additional factors that can contribute to obesity when cortisol levels are high.

Also, inadequate sleep may alter insulin sensitivity, which may result in a rise in blood sugar levels. Moreover, this may contribute to weight gain and raise the possibility of type 2 diabetes.

In general, getting too little sleep can have a negative effect on one's health and can contribute significantly to the onset of obesity. In order to lower the risk of obesity, it is crucial to make sure that appropriate amounts of high-quality sleep are attained.

Emotional components:

Obesity is often caused by emotional factors. Stress, despair, and other unfavorable emotions can cause overeating and make people make bad dietary decisions, which can result in weight gain and obesity. In an effort to deal with their feelings, people who are stressed may turn to comfort food or overeat. Stress is a primary contributor to overeating. In an effort to lift their spirits or to detach from unpleasant feelings, depressed people may also overeat.

Also, those who are emotionally weak may be more prone to using food as a kind of self-indulgence or as a way to "reward" themselves. Eating can become a coping mechanism for distressing feelings, developing into an unhealthy dependence on food. Last but not least, those who don't have enough social support may also be more inclined to overeat as a coping mechanism for loneliness or social isolation.

Overall, obesity might have a significant emotional component. Negative emotions such as stress, depression, and others can cause overeating, which can result in weight gain and obesity. In order to address these concerns, it is critical to acknowledge the contribution of emotional aspects to obesity and look for good coping strategies, such as exercise and talking to a trusted friend or counselor.

Understanding the origins and effects of obesity can help people, communities, and policymakers collaborate to lower the incidence of obesity and the health hazards it entails.

CHAPTER 2

EFFECTS OF OBESITY

Risks to health:

One of the biggest issues with public health in the current era is obesity. It is closely associated with a number of major health hazards, such as heart disease, diabetes, stroke, and several forms of cancer. This essay will go into great length about the health problems associated with obesity and give a general outline of how it can be prevented and treated.

To put it simply, obesity is essentially just having too much body fat. The typical method of determining it is to calculate a person's body mass index (BMI), which is a ratio of their weight in kilograms divided by the square of their height in meters. Obesity is defined as having a BMI of 30 or higher.

Obesity carries a host of health hazards. It can raise someone's chance of getting a number of chronic illnesses, such as heart disease, type 2 diabetes, stroke, and some types of cancer (e.g., breast, colon, and endometrial). The quality of life and lifespan of an individual may be significantly impacted by these disorders.

The most prevalent and dangerous health risk related to obesity is heart disease. This condition is brought on by an accumulation of fatty deposits in the arteries, which can result in a heart attack or stroke. Due to their greater amounts of body fat and cholesterol, obese people have a higher risk of developing heart disease.

An additional significant health concern linked to obesity is type 2 diabetes. It is a chronic disorder in which the body has difficulty metabolizing glucose, leading to elevated blood sugar levels. Because of their excess weight and fat, obese people have a higher chance of acquiring type 2 diabetes.

High blood pressure, sleep apnea, osteoarthritis, and some types of cancer are just a few of the health issues that obesity can cause. It may also result in psychological issues like depression, anxiety, and low self-esteem.

Together with it, there are additional health difficulties like osteoarthritis and gallbladder disease (a breakdown of cartilage and bone within a joint).

Respiratory issues and sleep apnea poor life quality, psychological problems such as clinical depression, anxiety, and others, physical dysfunction and discomfort in the body.

Economic effects of obesity:

There has been a major decline in physical activity and a global shift in food consumption habits toward meals that are higher in calories. Obese and overweight people have a much increased risk of developing non-communicable diseases.

Obesity has a significant negative influence on national economies by shortening lifespans, lowering productivity, and raising disability and medical expenses.

In 2016, there were more than 2 billion overweight or obese people in the world, and more than 70% of them lived in low- or middle-income nations.

With a high prevalence of both undernutrition and obesity, many low- and middle-income nations bear a double burden. Obesity becomes more prevalent among the poor and in rural regions as per capita income rises.

In terms of prevalence, incidence, and financial impact, obesity represents a significant threat to the health of the national and international population. In 2014, more than 2.1 billion people, or nearly 30% of the world's population, were overweight or obese, and obesity was a factor in 5% of global fatalities. In 2014, more than 2.1 billion people, or nearly 30% of the world's population, were overweight or obese, and obesity was a factor in 5% of global fatalities. By 2030, nearly half of all adults worldwide will be overweight or obese if the current incidence rate is maintained.

The economic costs of obesity are significant for the individual as well as for families, communities, and countries. The estimated cost of obesity to the world economy in 2014 was $2.0 trillion, or 2.8% of the global GDP (GDP). In addition to increased medical costs, obesity also has a negative impact on the economy due to lost workdays, decreased productivity at work, mortality, and permanent impairment. Several studies and analyses have noted that there is a gradient between rising BMI and the costs associated with obesity.

A peer-reviewed study published in BMJ Global Health estimates that the economic costs of overweight and obesity will climb from 2.19% to 3.3% of GDP in 161 countries.

According to the study, maintaining the global overweight and obesity incidence at 2019 levels would result in annual savings of US$2.2 trillion.

Low-resource nations would bear the brunt of the increase in GDP costs, which are anticipated to be 12–25 times higher than levels in 2019.

China (almost $10 trillion), the United States (over $2.5 trillion), and India (nearly $850 billion) are the nations likely to bear the heaviest economic burdens from overweight and obesity.

New York, September 21st, 2022 In 2060, the Global Obesity Federation and RTI International predict that the incidence of overweight and obesity will cost the world economy 3.3% of its GDP.

Obesity has become a serious global issue over the past few decades. More than two-thirds of persons in the US are overweight, and one third are obese. In this article, we give a summary of the current state of study on the potential national economic effects of the obesity epidemic in the US.

Direct medical expenditures, productivity costs, transportation costs, and human capital costs are the top four areas of economic effect currently associated with the obesity pandemic.

Direct medical spending is one of the most frequently mentioned negative economic effects of the obesity epidemic. Obesity raises the chance of developing a number of significant health diseases, including type 2 diabetes, coronary heart disease (CHD), stroke, asthma, and arthritis.

When obesity rates rise, direct medical spending on the identification and treatment of these disorders is consequently likely to rise. Several studies provide retrospective or prospective estimates of the frequency of diseases that can be connected to obesity as well as the scope of related direct medical expenses.

The indirect economic consequences of obesity include lost production as a result of disease and early death, as well as expenses related to absenteeism and presenteeism, which is when a worker is present at work but is less productive owing to illness.

Together with these direct and indirect expenses, there are also expenses related to the stigma and prejudice suffered by those who are obese. Reduced self-esteem, trouble locating a job or a place to live, and an elevated risk of depression are all consequences of stigma and prejudice. These psychological impacts may further reduce productivity and raise the cost of healthcare.

CHAPTER 3
OBESITY TREATMENT AND PREVENTION

Exercise and diet: Because of your gradual weight gain, a family history of obesity, a health condition that is associated with obesity, or even simply a general concern for maintaining your health, you may be worried about preventing obesity. Whatever your motivation, the objective is deserving.

Avoiding obesity lowers your chance of a variety of related health problems, including heart disease, diabetes, some cancers, and a lot of other conditions.

Similar to many other chronic disorders, obesity can be avoided by leading a healthy lifestyle that includes regular exercise, wholesome food, enough sleep, and other activities. The treatment tactics are the same as the preventative measures if you are already overweight or obese.

By adhering to the fundamentals of good eating, obesity can be avoided. These are some easy dietary adjustments you may adopt to aid with weight loss and prevent obesity.

Take five servings of fruit and vegetables each day. Always strive to get five to seven servings of whole fruits and veggies daily. Low-calorie foods include fruits and vegetables. According to the WHO, there is strong proof that consuming fruits and vegetables lowers the risk of becoming obese.

They have higher nutritional concentrations and are linked to a lower incidence of insulin resistance and diabetes. Its high fiber content in particular makes you feel full on fewer calories, assisting in weight loss.

Eat unprocessed food instead: Empty calories are a typical source and can pile up quickly in highly processed meals like white bread and in many packed snacks. In a 2019 study, it was discovered that participants fed a highly processed diet ingested more calories and put on weight, whereas those offered a less processed diet consumed fewer calories and shed pounds.

Limit your intake of added sugars:

It's critical to limit your intake of added sugars. The American Heart Association advises men and women to consume no more than six teaspoons of added sugar daily, respectively. The main added sugar sources to avoid include sweetened beverages, such as soda and energy or sports drinks; sweetened grains like pies, cookies, and cakes; fruit drinks (which are rarely 100% fruit juice); candies; and dairy desserts like ice cream.

Avoid using artificial sweeteners: Artificial sweeteners have been connected to diabetes and obesity. Use a small bit of honey as a natural option if you feel the need to use a sweetener.

Avoid saturated fats: According to a 2018 study, eating foods high in saturated fats causes obesity.

Instead, pay attention to foods like avocados, olive oil, and tree nuts that are good providers of mono- and polyunsaturated fats. Even good fats should only make up

20% to 35% of daily calories, and individuals with high cholesterol or vascular disease may require even less.

Be careful what you drink: Increase your water intake, and do away with any sugar-sweetened beverages. Use water as your primary beverage; unsweetened tea and coffee are also acceptable. Avoid energy and sports drinks, which not only contain excessive amounts of added sugar but also may be harmful to your cardiovascular system (in the case of the former).

Domestic cooking Men and women who regularly prepare meals at home are less likely to gain weight, according to studies that examined this topic. Type 2 diabetes was also less likely to strike them.

Give a plant-based diet a shot. An increase in general health and a significantly reduced incidence of obesity have been linked to eating a plant-based diet. Fill as much of your plate as possible with whole fruits and vegetables to achieve this. Consume tiny amounts (about 1.5 ounces or a small handful) of unsalted nuts for snacks. These include almonds, cashews, walnuts, and pistachios, all of which are good for your heart. Reduce your intake of protein sources that are high in saturated fats, such as red meat and dairy, or cut them out entirely.

Exercise:

According to the majority of national and international guidelines, an average adult should engage in 150 minutes per week of moderate-intensity exercise. For five days a week, that translates to at least 30 minutes per day.

Brisk walking is the best exercise for keeping a healthy weight, according to a study of the 2015 Health Survey for England data.

In comparison to people engaging in other activities, researchers discovered that people who walk quickly or briskly are more likely to be lighter, have a lower body mass index (BMI), and have smaller waists.

Also, experts advise staying active all day long, whether by adopting a standing desk, taking frequent stretch breaks, or finding methods to incorporate walking meetings into your schedule.

HOW TO LOSE WEIGHT

1. Ensure that you're prepared

Long-term weight loss requires patience, hard work, and dedication. Although you shouldn't put off losing weight permanently, you should make sure you're prepared to make lasting changes to your food and exercise routine. To assess your preparation, pose the following questions to yourself:

- Is weight loss motivating me?
- Am I being too distracted by other obligations?
- Do I use food as a coping mechanism for stress?
- Am I prepared to learn or employ additional stress management techniques?
- Do I require more assistance managing my stress, such as from friends or professionals?
- Am I prepared to alter my eating habits?
- Am I willing to alter my exercise routine?
- Will I have enough time to devote to making these changes?

If circumstances or emotions seem to be impeding your readiness, talk to your doctor if you need assistance. Setting goals, maintaining commitment, and altering behaviors will be simpler for you when you're ready.

2.   Discover your internal motivation.

Nobody else is able to force you to lose weight. For your own satisfaction, you must make dietary and activity modifications. What will provide you with the impetus to follow through on your weight-loss plan?

If you want to stay motivated and focused, make a list of your top priorities, such as a future trip or improved general health. Once you've done that, figure out how to make sure you can use your motivating elements when you're tempted. You may, for instance, write a motivating note to yourself on the refrigerator or pantry door.

For successful weight loss, you must be accountable for your own actions, but it also helps to have the proper type of support. Choose supporters who will motivate you positively and free of guilt, embarrassment, or sabotage.

Find friends who will ideally listen to your worries and emotions, spend time working out with you or preparing healthy meals, and share the importance you place on leading a healthier lifestyle. Accountability provided by your support group can be a powerful incentive to remain committed to your weight-loss objectives.

If you'd rather keep your weight-loss ambitions a secret, hold yourself accountable by regularly checking your weight, keeping track of your diet and exercise efforts in a notebook, or monitoring your success with digital tools.

3. Make sensible objectives.

Setting realistic weight-loss targets might seem obvious. But do you actually understand what is realistic? Aiming to lose 1 to 2 pounds (0.5 to 1 kilogram) per week is a wise long-term strategy. With a reduced-calorie diet and consistent exercise, you may typically lose 1 to 2 pounds each week by burning 500 to 1,000 more calories than you take in.

5% of your present weight may be a reasonable objective, at least as a first aim, depending on your weight. If you are 180 pounds, that is 9 pounds (82 kilos) (4 kilograms). Even a small amount of weight loss can reduce your risk of developing long-term health issues like type 2 diabetes and heart disease.

Consider both process and end goals as you define your objectives. A process objective may be "Walk for 30 minutes each day." A sample result target is "Lose 10 pounds." Although altering your habits is the key to losing weight, having an outcome objective is not necessary. Instead, you should develop process goals.

4. Consume wholesome food.

You must reduce your overall calorie consumption when changing your eating habits to support weight loss. Yet, cutting calories doesn't have to entail sacrificing flavor, satisfaction, or even convenience in the kitchen.

Eating more plant-based foods, such as whole grains, fruits, and vegetables, is one approach to reducing your calorie intake. To attain your goals without sacrificing nutrition or taste, strive for variety.

Follow this advice to begin losing weight:

- Consume at least three servings of fruit and four servings of veggies each day.
- Rather than processed grains, choose whole grains.
- Use little amounts of healthy fats such as avocados, nuts, nut butters, olive oil, vegetable oils, and nut oils.
- Apart from the natural sugar in fruit, reduce your intake of sugar as much as you can.
- Choose restricted amounts of lean meat and poultry and low-fat dairy products.

5. Be active and keep active.

Although you can lose weight without exercising, combining calorie restriction with regular physical activity can offer you an advantage. The extra calories you couldn't lose with food alone can be burned off with exercise.

Also, exercise has several positive health effects, such as elevating your mood, enhancing your cardiovascular system, and lowering your blood pressure. Maintaining weight loss can also be aided by exercise. According to studies, those who are able to keep off their weight in the long run engage in regular physical activity.

The frequency, length, and intensity of your exercises will determine how many calories you burn. Consistent aerobic activity for at least 30 minutes most days of the week, such as brisk walking, is one of the greatest strategies to shed body fat. To lose weight and keep it off, some people might need to engage in more physical activity than this.

Every additional exercise helps burn calories. If you are unable to squeeze in formal exercise on a particular day, consider ways you might improve your physical activity throughout the day. For instance, park at the far end of the parking lot when you're shopping or make multiple trips up and down the stairs rather than taking the elevator.

6. Modify your outlook

If you want long-term, effective weight management, it is not enough to eat healthily and exercise for only a few weeks or even months. These routines must be adopted as a way of life. The first step in making lifestyle changes is to examine your daily schedule and eating habits honestly.

After evaluating your specific obstacles, consider developing a plan to progressively alter the behaviors and mindsets that have undermined your prior attempts at weight loss. If you want to be successful in your efforts to lose weight permanently, go beyond simply acknowledging your obstacles and make a plan for how you'll overcome them.

You'll probably experience setbacks every so often. Yet after a setback, just start over the following day instead of completely giving up. Do not forget that you want to alter your life. That won't occur all at once. The outcomes will be worthwhile if you maintain your healthy lifestyle.

7. Medical Interventions:

Millions of people all over the world struggle to maintain a healthy weight, making obesity a significant health concern in today's culture. Obesity can cause heart disease, type 2 diabetes, stroke, and other illnesses. It can also hasten the aging process. Fortunately, there are many treatments available to aid with weight management and health improvement.

I. Appetite suppressant: One such treatment option that can be utilized to lower caloric consumption and assist people in reaching their ideal weight is appetite suppressants.

Medicines known as appetite suppressants are intended to lessen desires and hunger, which will lower how much food a person eats. They fall into two categories: prescription drugs, which are governed by the Food and Drug Administration (FDA), and over-the-counter supplements, which are not. Both kinds of appetite suppressants function by focusing on various brain and body regions to lessen cravings, decrease hunger, and boost the sense of fullness after eating.

Patients who are extremely obese or who have trouble controlling their food intake typically benefit from using prescription appetite suppressants, which are typically given by a doctor. Phentermine, a stimulant that works, is the most popular prescription appetite suppressor.

II. Anti-lipase agents

Drugs called lipase inhibitors prevent the enzymes called lipases from breaking down dietary lipids. Lipase inhibitors reduce the amount of calories that are absorbed by the body by inhibiting the action of lipases, which prevents the digestion of dietary fats.

Lipase inhibitors are frequently given before meals while being used to treat obesity. The drug binds to the lipase enzymes in the gastrointestinal tract and stops them from metabolizing dietary fats. By not being digested, the fats pass through the digestive system, lowering the amount of calories that are ingested.

In addition to decreasing hunger, lipase inhibitors can aid weight loss efforts. Lipase inhibitors can lessen the sense of fullness a person has after eating because they prevent the absorption of dietary lipids. The reduction in total calorie intake, a crucial element of any effective weight loss plan, might be made easier for people as a result.

Lipase inhibitors are able to improve triglyceride levels, which are crucial for preserving a healthy weight, in addition to decreasing calorie absorption and hunger. Triglycerides are a form of fat that can raise the risk of heart disease and stroke, so using lipase inhibitors to lower them can be beneficial for overall health.

Combination medicine: Combination medicine is a type of obesity treatment in which two or more medications are combined to create a more potent treatment for obesity. Combination drugs function by focusing on many facets of obesity, including appetite suppression, fat metabolism, and energy expenditure.

Combinations of an appetite suppressant, like Phentermine, and an anti-lipase prescription, like Orlistat, are the most frequently prescribed treatments for obesity. While the anti-lipase medication helps stop the body from absorbing and storing fat from the food you eat, the appetite suppressant aids in reducing hunger cravings and encourages the body to burn stored fat for energy.

These two drugs, taken together, have the potential to be very successful in reducing extra body fat. While the anti-lipase medication helps to stop the body from absorbing and storing fat from the food you eat, the appetite suppressant aids in reducing hunger cravings. This aids in lowering calorie intake overall and stimulates the body to burn stored fat for energy.

Combination drugs also aid in lowering cravings for unhealthy meals, which may aid in lowering total calorie consumption. For people who find it difficult to curb their appetites and cravings for unhealthy meals, this can be very helpful.

Moreover, a combination of medications may help to increase energy expenditure and metabolism. This promotes increased calorie burn throughout the day and stimulates the body to utilize fat reserves for energy.

Overall, a combination of medications can be a highly successful way to treat obesity. It can aid in reducing total body fat and enhancing health by focusing on various facets of obesity, including appetite suppression, fat metabolism, and energy expenditure.

SURGERY:

The main medical method used to treat obesity is surgery. By reducing the quantity of food, the stomach can hold or by changing the intestine so that fewer calories are absorbed, it works. When other weight-loss strategies, like diet and exercise, have failed, surgery is typically regarded as a last resort.

Gastric bypass surgery is the most popular procedure for treating obesity. Making a little stomach pouch and joining it to the small intestine directly are the steps in this method. As a result, the person can consume less food and must eat until they are full. The body has a tougher time absorbing calories from food as a result.

Gastric banding is an additional procedure used to manage obesity. In this method, a band that may be adjusted for tightness or looseness is wrapped around the top of the stomach for tightness or looseness is wrapped around the top of the stomach. By limiting how much food a person can consume, this can help them lose weight.

Together with the surgeries mentioned above, there are other procedures including stomach stapling and biliopancreatic diversion. These more difficult procedures are often only employed in the most severe forms of obesity.

Before making any decisions, patients should explore all the risks of surgery with their doctor. Surgery is a serious medical operation. It is crucial to keep in mind that surgery is not a quick fix and that maintaining a healthy lifestyle through food and exercise is necessary to keep the weight off. Although it should always be evaluated in conjunction with other weight-loss strategies, surgery can be a useful treatment for obesity.

CHAPTER 4

CONCLUSION

The extensive examination of the causes of obesity in this book has underlined the need for a multifaceted strategy to prevent and address this pressing worldwide health problem. However, it also emphasized the need for other factors, like environmental and socioeconomic factors, to be taken into consideration when considering obesity prevention strategies. Lifestyle interventions, such as healthy eating and increased physical activity, have been discussed as being important. The necessity of improved public health awareness, the function of the healthcare system in resolving the issue, and the necessity of a multi-sectoral strategy to do so have also been covered.

It has emphasized the necessity of quick action to stop the obesity epidemic from spreading further as well as the significance of cooperation among diverse stakeholders, including health care providers, community organizations, and policy makers. It is crucial for individuals, families, and communities to collaborate in order to foster a supportive atmosphere and guarantee that everyone has access to the necessary tools in order to successfully prevent and manage obesity in the future.

The book shed light on the complexity of the obesity epidemic and emphasized the need to take into account all factors in order to address the issue in a meaningful way. It has given medical professionals a useful resource.